HOW TO GET FIT UNDER AN HOUR A DAY

SIMPLE ONE HOUR EXERCISE PLAN FOR A NOVICE

CYRIL LAKES

Contents

CHAPTER ONE

INTRODUCTION

It might be difficult to find time for fitness in the fast-paced world of today. It is easy to feel as though there is simply not enough time in the day to prioritize exercising with work, family, and other obligations. Nevertheless, staying in shape doesn't have to include lengthy workouts or rigorous regimens. You may reach your fitness objectives in less than an hour every day if you have the proper strategy and are dedicated to consistency.

We'll go over doable tactics and productive exercises in this article to help you maintain your health and fitness levels despite a hectic schedule. This guide will provide you the skills and inspiration to maximize your time and produce long-lasting effects, whether you're a novice trying to start a fitness regimen or an experienced athlete looking for effective routines.

We'll explore a range of workout alternatives that may be customized to your fitness level and tastes, from bodyweight exercises to high-intensity interval training (HIIT). Along the way, we'll talk about how crucial it is to support your fitness journey and optimize your outcomes with appropriate nutrition, hydration, and recovery.

You have the ability to take charge of your health and wellbeing regardless of your age, level of fitness, or schedule constraints. Even a small portion of your day can be spent exercising to increase your strength, stamina, and general quality of life. In less than an hour a day, let's begin the journey to a better, more fit version of ourselves.

Exercise's importance for mental and physical health

Promoting both physical and emotional well-being requires regular exercise. This is the reason it's critical for general health:

Advantages for Physical Health:

Enhances Cardiovascular Health: Frequent exercise lowers the risk of high blood pressure, heart disease, and stroke by strengthening the heart and improving circulation.

Strengthens Bones and Muscles: By increasing bone density and strengthening muscles, weight-bearing activities lower the risk of osteoporosis and fractures.

Helps with Weight Management: When paired with a nutritious diet, exercise can aid with weight loss or maintenance by burning calories and increasing lean muscle mass.

Boosts Immune Function: Engaging in regular physical activity fortifies the immune system, lowering the risk of disease and fostering resilience and general health.

Enhances Chronic Disease Management: By easing symptoms and lowering consequences, exercise can aid in the management and prevention of chronic illnesses like diabetes, rheumatoid arthritis, and some forms of cancer.

Advantages for Mental Health:

Reduces tension and Anxiety: Engaging in physical activity causes the body to produce endorphins, which are neurotransmitters that aid in reducing tension and anxiety and fostering a feeling of wellbeing.

Enhances Mood and Happiness: Dopamine and serotonin, two neurotransmitters that are linked to emotions of pleasure and happiness, are released during exercise. Frequent exercise can lessen depressive symptoms and elevate mood.

Enhances Cognitive Function: By boosting blood flow to the brain and encouraging the development of new neurons, aerobic exercise enhances memory, cognitive function, and brain function.

Encourages Better Sleep: Frequent exercise can help control sleep cycles and enhance the quality of sleep, which will improve slumber and give you more energy during the day.

Builds Resilience to Mental Health Challenges: Physical activity promotes resilience and emotional well-being by offering a healthy coping strategy for handling stress, sorrow, and other mental health issues.

General Well-Being:

Boosts Energy and Vitality: By increasing circulation, oxygenation, and metabolism, exercise increases energy levels and lessens symptoms of exhaustion.

Increases Self-Esteem and Confidence: Reaching fitness objectives and bettering one's physical condition can increase one's sense of self-worth and self-assurance, which can result in a higher sense of body acceptance and contentment.

Encourages Social Connection: Taking part in sports or group fitness programs can encourage social contact, collaboration, and a sense of belonging, which can lessen feelings of isolation and loneliness.

Engaging in physical exercise is an effective way to support mental and physical health. You may raise your quality of life, lower your risk of chronic disease, and improve your general health by including regular physical activity in your routine. Exercise may become a fulfilling and lasting part of your life by finding things you enjoy, whether it's going for a walk, working out at the gym, or doing yoga.

Creating Reasonable Fitness Objectives

In order to be consistent, stay inspired, and succeed long-term in your fitness journey, you must set reasonable fitness goals. You can set reasonable fitness goals by following these steps:

Determine Your present Fitness Level: To begin, determine your present level of fitness, taking into account your advantages, disadvantages, and potential growth areas. Take into account elements like your body composition, strength, flexibility, and cardiovascular endurance.

Establish Your Priorities: Choose the aspects of exercise and health that are most important to you. Are you concentrating on enhancing your general well-being, decreasing body weight, gaining muscle, boosting stamina, or reaching particular sporting objectives? You can create goals that are consistent with your values and aspirations by making your priorities clear.

Establish Clear, Specific, Measurable Goals: To monitor your progress and maintain accountability, clearly define, measure, and monitor your goals. Set precise objectives like "run a 5K race in under 30 minutes" or "lose 10 pounds in three months" in place of general ones like "get in shape" or "lose weight."

Divide Your Objectives: Divide more ambitious objectives into more manageable benchmarks. This lessens their intimidating nature and enables you to acknowledge your accomplishments as you go. If your objective is to run a marathon, for instance, establish intermediate targets like finishing a 10K race or a half marathon.

Be Attainable and Realistic: Based on your existing resources, lifestyle, and fitness level, set challenging but realistic goals. Steer clear of overly ambitious aspirations since they could cause dissatisfaction or fatigue. Think about things like your age, past fitness levels, free time, and any restrictions or limits.

Set a Timeline: Determine a reasonable amount of time that will allow you to accomplish your objectives, accounting for your starting place, your rate of advancement, and any outside influences that might affect your course. To help you stay on course, divide your timeframe into short-, medium-, and long-term goals.

Think About SMART Criteria: Make sure your objectives are time-bound, relevant, quantifiable, specified, and achievable by using the SMART criteria. You can set more successful and clearly defined goals with the aid of this framework.

Adapt as Necessary: Remain adaptable and prepared to modify your objectives in light of your development, evolving circumstances, and physical input. If you run into difficulties or your priorities change over time, don't be afraid to adjust your goals.

Celebrate Your Successes: No matter how tiny, acknowledge and appreciate your victories and accomplishments along the road. To maintain motivation and focus on your objectives, utilize positive reinforcement, acknowledge your progress, and reward yourself when you meet milestones.

Remain Patient and Consistent: Long-term success in reaching your fitness objectives requires consistency. Even when it seems like development is taking a while, don't waver from your exercise regimen, diet, and recuperation techniques. Remind yourself to be patient with yourself, trust the process, and keep in mind that lasting change requires time and work.

You may make a clear plan for your fitness journey and improve your chances of success by following these steps and creating reasonable fitness goals. In order to become the healthiest and happiest version of yourself, never lose concentration or motivation.

CHAPTER TWO

Organizing Your Exercise

To reach your fitness objectives, maximize efficiency, and maintain motivation, you must plan your workouts. You may efficiently schedule your workouts by following these steps:

Establish Your Objectives: To begin, identify your fitness objectives. Are you trying to increase your flexibility, decrease weight, gain strength, or gain better endurance? Your workout planning approach will be guided by your understanding of your goals.

Determine Your Present Fitness Level: Determine your present level of fitness, taking into account your advantages, disadvantages, and potential growth areas. Take into account elements like body composition, muscular strength, flexibility, and cardiovascular endurance.

Establish a Well-Balanced Program: Formulate a comprehensive fitness program that incorporates a variety of cardio-vascular exercises, weight training, flexibility exercises, and recovery days. To minimize overuse injuries and boredom, strive for variation.

Think About Frequency and Duration: Choose the number of times per week you'll work out and the length of each session. Strive for equilibrium between pushing yourself to the limit and giving yourself enough time to heal. As your fitness level rises, gradually increase the intensity, frequency, and duration.

Choose Exercises and hobbies You Enjoy: Make sure your workouts and hobbies are something you look forward to. Exercise becomes more pleasurable and more adherence-boosting when you choose activities you love, whether it's dance, yoga, weightlifting, cycling, jogging, or swimming.

Have Reasonable Expectations: Be honest with yourself about your ability to improve both now and in the future. Based on your present fitness level, availability, and timetable, set realistic goals. Steer clear of overcommitting or establishing unattainable goals, as they can result in disappointment or burnout.

Plan for Progression: Gradually increase the duration, intensity, or complexity of your exercises over time to incorporate progressive overload into your workouts. This encourages adaptation and guarantees that you'll keep moving closer to your fitness objectives.

Plan Your Workouts: Set aside specific times in your weekly plan for your workouts. Consider these self-care appointments as unchangeable obligations and arrange them in order of importance. The secret to getting results is consistency.

Listen to Your Body: Observe how your body feels both during and following exercise. Adapt your workout to your current level of intensity, volume, or choice of exercises, and pay attention to any symptoms of overtraining, soreness, or exhaustion.

Plan for Recovery: To give your body enough time to heal and rebuild, including active recovery exercises and rest days into your training regimen. To aid with your recuperation, put an emphasis on healthy eating, staying hydrated, getting enough sleep, and managing stress.

Track Your Progress: To keep track of your workouts, chart your progress, and see how much you've improved over time, keep a workout journal or use a fitness tracking app. Honor accomplishments, no matter how tiny, and turn failures into teaching moments.

Be Adaptable: Be ready to modify your exercise regimen as necessary to account for shifts in your preferences, schedule, or situation. Retaining consistency and adjusting to the unpredictable nature of life require flexibility.

In order to achieve your fitness goals, you can maximize your time, effort, and results by following these guidelines and arranging your workouts strategically. Remain dedicated, keep inspired, and relish the process of becoming a stronger, healthier, and happier version of yourself.

Getting the Most Out of Your Time

Prioritization and strategic planning are necessary to maximize the amount of time that may be spent exercising in an hour. The following advice will help you maximize the time you spend working out:

Establish Specific Objectives: Ascertain the desired outcomes for your exercise regimen. You can choose and intensify your exercises based on certain goals, such as burning calories, strengthening your cardiovascular system, or enhancing your strength.

Put an emphasis on Compound Exercises: Select multi-joint, compound exercises that work several muscle groups at once. Squats, deadlifts, lunges, push-ups, pull-ups, and rows are a few examples. Compound exercises are a great way to increase muscle mass and burn calories quickly.

Add in High-Intensity Interval Training (HIIT): HIIT alternates brief rest intervals with short bursts of vigorous activity. It's a quick and effective approach to increase metabolism, burn calories, and enhance cardiovascular fitness. Think about incorporating HIIT exercises into your program, like burpees, jumping jacks, sprints, or cycling intervals.

Superset Strength Exercises: To optimize time efficiency and boost workout intensity, pair two or more strength exercises back-to-back with little to no rest in between sets. For instance, switch up your lower and upper body workouts, or focus on opposing muscle regions (like your back and chest).

Reduce Rest Time: To maintain a high heart rate and optimize calorie burn, reduce the amount of time you rest in between sets and activities. For strength training activities, aim for 30 to 60 seconds of rest in between sets; for HIIT intervals, aim for shorter rest times.

Employ Circuit Training: Circuit training entails carrying out a set of exercises one after the other with little to no break in between. Create a circuit that alternates between cardiovascular and strength training, and move swiftly between exercises to maintain an elevated heart rate and maximum burning of calories.

Optimize Your Cardiovascular Workouts: Pick cardiovascular exercises that offer the best cardiovascular and calorie-burning value.

Exercises that maximize calorie expenditure in a brief period of time include running, cycling, rowing, and jump rope.

Prepare Your Workouts Ahead of Time: Before you begin your session, have a well-organized training schedule in place. This will enable you to maximize your time at home or in the gym by maintaining focus. To hold yourself accountable, record your workouts, sets, repetitions, and rest times in writing.

Drink water before, during, and after your workout to stay hydrated and fuel your body for maximum performance. Before your workout, fuel your body with a balanced lunch or snack that includes both protein and carbs to enhance muscle repair and give you energy.

Cool Down and Stretch: After your workout, set aside some time for a quick stretch and cooldown. This lowers heart rate, avoids discomfort in the muscles, and increases range of motion and flexibility.

You can do an intense workout in under an hour if you put these methods into practice and make the most of every minute of your workout. To get the most out of your workouts and move closer to your fitness objectives, keep in mind that intensity, consistency, and good form come first.

Making Cardiovascular Exercise a Priority

Making cardiovascular exercise a priority in a one-hour workout regimen calls for organization and efficiency. Here's how to plan your workout to get the most cardiovascular benefits in this amount of time:

Five minutes for warm-up:

Warm up for a short while to get your body ready for workout. Include dynamic exercises to raise heart rate, loosen muscles, and develop flexibility, such as arm circles, leg swings, running in place, or jumping jacks.

30- to 35-minute Main Cardiovascular Workout:

Select a vigorous cardiovascular exercise that makes use of your major muscle groups and raises your heart rate. Choices consist of:

Jogging or running outside or using a treadmill

Riding a stationary bike or going outside

Using a rowing machine to row

Rope jumping

workouts using high-intensity interval training (HIIT) that include aerobic activities including burpees, sprints, and mountain climbers

Plan your cardiovascular exercise such that you alternate between times of increased intensity and active recovery. For instance, switch off between one minute of moderate effort (like walking or running) and one minute of intensive effort (like sprinting).

Exercise for Strength (15–20 minutes):

Although cardiovascular exercise takes precedence, adding strength training to your regimen can enhance your general health and offer extra advantages. Pay attention to compound workouts that work several muscular groups, like:

Bodyweight workouts such as planks, squats, lunges, and push-ups

Exercises with dumbbells or kettlebells, such as lunges, pushes, rows, and deadlifts

Resistance band workouts to build strength in the upper and lower body

For each exercise, do 2-3 sets of 8–12 repetitions, taking little to no break in between sets to maintain a raised heart rate.

Stretch and cool down for five to ten minutes:

Spend some time cooling down and stretching your muscles after your strength and aerobic workouts. Stretch your major muscle groups static, holding each pose for 15–30 seconds to increase flexibility and lower your chance of injury.

During your workout, pay particular attention to the muscles in your legs, back, chest, and shoulders.

Rehydration and Hydration:

Water should be consumed prior to, during, and after exercise to help you stay hydrated. Resupply electrolytes if you've been perspiring a lot.

After your workout, give yourself enough time to recover properly. This includes nourishing your body with a balanced breakfast or snack that includes both protein and carbohydrates to aid in muscle regeneration and restore energy reserves.

You may optimize your calorie burn, enhance your cardiovascular fitness, and enjoy the many health advantages of regular aerobic exercise by making cardiovascular exercise a priority in your one-hour workout schedule and including effective, high-intensity exercises. Based on your fitness level, objectives, and personal preferences, modify the intensity and length of your workout. Also, don't forget to pay attention to your body and make any adjustments.

Including Strength Training

Including strength training in your one-hour workout regimen calls for productivity and concentration. Here's how to plan your workout so that it includes efficient strength training in this amount of time:

Five minutes for warm-up:

Warm up for a short while to improve blood flow to your muscles and get your body ready for exercise. To release tension in your joints and muscles, try dynamic exercises like bodyweight squats, shoulder circles, arm circles, and leg swings.

Exercise for Strength (30–35 minutes):

To achieve maximum efficiency and efficacy, concentrate on complex workouts that engage many muscle groups simultaneously. Select a range of exercises that target various body parts, such as:

Squats: Work the quadriceps, hamstrings, and glutes, among other lower body muscles.

Deadlifts: These exercises target the lower back, hamstrings, and glutes as well as the posterior chain.

Using the triceps, shoulders, and chest, perform a bench press.

Strengthening the shoulders, biceps, and back with pull-ups or rows.

Overhead Press: This exercise works the upper back, triceps, and shoulders.

Lunges: These exercises strengthen the legs and glutes while enhancing stability and balance.

Work out three to four sets of eight to twelve repetitions for each exercise, using a weight that challenges you but doesn't compromise form.

To maintain a raised heart rate and optimize calorie burn, minimize downtime in between sessions.

Exercise for the Heart (15–20 minutes):

To further boost calorie expenditure and enhance cardiovascular fitness, switch from strength training to aerobic exercise after your workout.

Select a vigorous aerobic exercise, such as:

Jogging or running outside or on a treadmill

Riding a stationary bike or going outside

Using a rowing machine to row

Rope jumping

Mountain climbers, burpees, and sprints are examples of cardio exercises included in high-intensity interval training (HIIT).

To maintain a raised heart rate and optimize cardiovascular benefits, alternate periods of intense exercise with active rest.

Stretch and cool down for five to ten minutes:

Stretching and a cool-down after your workout will increase your flexibility, lessen discomfort in your muscles, and speed up your recuperation.

Stretching should be concentrated on, with each stretch held for 15–30 seconds, the muscles you worked during your strength training and cardio workout.

Give special attention to the muscles in your chest, shoulders, back, hamstrings, quadriceps, and calves as these are particularly prone to injury or tightness.

Rehydration and Hydration:

Be sure to stay hydrated by drinking water prior to, during, and after your workout. Resupply electrolytes if you've been perspiring a lot.

After your workout, give yourself enough time to recover properly. This includes nourishing your body with a balanced breakfast or snack that includes both protein and carbohydrates to aid in muscle regeneration and restore energy reserves.

Strength training can help you achieve a well-rounded workout that supports your overall health and fitness goals by helping you gain muscle mass, enhance cardiovascular fitness, and build strength during your one-hour exercise plan in addition to aerobic exercise. Depending on your fitness level, objectives, and personal preferences, change the volume and intensity of your workout. Also, don't forget to pay attention to your body and make any necessary adjustments.

Combining Mobility and Flexibility Training

For better joint health, injury prevention, and general movement quality, incorporate flexibility and mobility training into your one-hour workout routine. Here's how to plan your workout so that it includes efficient mobility and flexibility exercises in this amount of time:

Five minutes for warm-up:

To enhance blood flow, elevate pulse rate, and prime your muscles and joints for activity, begin your workout with a vigorous warm-up. Incorporate exercises that focus on important regions like the ankles, spine, shoulders, and hips. Trunk rotations, hip circles, leg swings, and arm circles are a few examples.

Movement Activities (10–15 minutes):

To increase joint flexibility and range of motion, engage in a series of mobility exercises. Pay attention to bodily parts including the hips, shoulders, ankles, and thoracic spine (upper back) that are prone to tightness or restriction. Incorporate mobility and stability-focused movements.

CHAPTER THREE

Examples of mobility drills are as follows:

Hip openers include pigeon position, hip circles, and hip flexor stretches.

Thoracic Spine Mobility: Thoracic extension using a foam roller, thoracic rotations, and the Cat-Cow stretch.

Shoulder Mobility: Wall slides, shoulder dislocations, and shoulder circles.

Ankle mobility exercises include dorsiflexion mobilizations, ankle circles, and calf stretches.

Exercises for Flexibility (10–15 minutes):

Include static stretching exercises to increase muscle length and flexibility. These muscles may be shortened or tight from extended sitting or repetitive motions. Stretches should be held for 15 to 30 seconds, with an emphasis on deep breathing and letting go of tension.

Aim for the major muscular groups in your body, such as your back, shoulders, chest, hamstrings, quadriceps, and calves.

Examples of exercises to improve flexibility are:

Stretching your hamstrings while standing

Stretching your quadriceps

Stretching the calf

Stretching your hip flexors

Stretching the chest opener

Stretch your shoulders

Cardiovascular or strength training (25–30 minutes):

Depending on your goals and preferences, move on to strength training or cardiovascular activity after finishing your flexibility and mobility work.

If your goal is strength training, use compound exercises that use your whole range of motion and focus on several muscle groups. Incorporate movements like lunges, rows, presses, pull-ups, deadlifts, and squats.

If you choose to exercise your heart, choose aerobic activities like swimming, cycling, rowing, or running that use a variety of joints and muscle groups and incorporate dynamic movement patterns.

Recovery and Cooling Off (5–10 minutes):

To reduce your heart rate and aid in recuperation, take a brief rest after your workout. After engaging in mild cardiovascular exercise, such as jogging or walking, stretch your major muscle groups static.

To assist your body in entering a state of healing and repair, concentrate on deep breathing and relaxation.

You may strengthen overall movement quality, lower your chance of injury, and improve joint health by adding flexibility and mobility training to your hour-long workout regimen. To guarantee correct form and technique, listen to your body and modify the time and intensity of your flexibility and mobility exercises based on your unique demands. Regularly performing mobility and flexibility exercises will eventually enhance range of motion, posture, and physical performance.

Developing a Daily Fitness Habit

Developing a daily routine of exercising is a great approach to put your health and wellbeing first. The following actions will assist you in creating and keeping up a regular exercise schedule:

Establish Clearly Defined, Measurable, Achievable Fitness Goals that Inspire You and Complement Your Values. Having specific goals gives your daily workouts direction and purpose, whether your objectives are to improve general fitness, lose weight, improve cardiovascular health, or increase strength.

Start Small: Set small, achievable fitness objectives that fit into your everyday schedule. As your endurance and confidence grow, progressively increase the amount of time and intensity of your daily exercise from the initial 10 to 15 minutes.

Plan Your Workouts: Put exercise on your daily schedule and treat it like an appointment that cannot be missed. Whether it's first thing in the morning, over your lunch break, or later in the evening after work, decide on a regular time of day that suits you best. You're more likely to maintain your fitness regimen if you prioritize it and set aside time for it.

Identify Pleasurable Activities: Opt for pursuits and workouts that you sincerely relish and eagerly anticipate. Finding activities you enjoy doing, whether it be weight training, cycling, swimming, dancing, yoga, or jogging, boosts motivation and makes it simpler to maintain your fitness regimen over time.

Mix It Up: Use a variety of exercises, activities, and training forms to keep your workouts fresh and engaging. To keep your body challenged and avoid boredom, alternate between cardiovascular activity, weight training, flexibility work, and leisure pursuits.

Have Reasonable Expectations: Be honest with yourself about your ability to improve both now and in the future. Based on your present fitness level, availability, and timetable, set attainable goals. Refrain from overcommitting or having irrational expectations as these might cause irritation or burnout.

Monitor Your Progress: To stay accountable and inspired, keep a record of your workouts, advancements, and accomplishments. Utilize a wearable fitness tracker, smartphone app, or fitness notebook to chart your workouts, keep tabs on your activity levels, and recognize your progress.

Make it Social: To make fitness more pleasurable and social, work out with friends, family, or fellow athletes. Join sports teams, online groups, or group fitness classes to meet like-minded people and maintain motivation through support and encouragement from one another.

Reward Yourself: Create a system of incentives to commemorate your fitness benchmarks and successes. After you accomplish a goal, treat yourself to something you appreciate, like a massage, a nutritious meal, or a new wardrobe for your workout. Incentives for continuous improvement and positive reinforcement can be found in rewards.

Remain Consistent: Developing a regular habit of exercise requires consistency. Make a commitment to being active, even if it's just for a quick walk or a few minutes of stretching, even on the days when you don't feel like it. Over time, consistency strengthens and accelerates the habit of regular exercise.

You can reap the many advantages of an active lifestyle as well as enhance your physical and mental well-being by following these guidelines and incorporating exercise into your everyday routine. Keep in mind that every little step matters and that working out helps you get closer to your objectives.

Maximizing Nutrient Intake for Exercise

Sustaining your fitness objectives and getting the most out of your efforts depend on optimizing your diet. Here's how to customize your diet to assist recuperation, fuel your exercises, and improve your general fitness:

Give macronutrients priority:

Protein: Protein is necessary for both the growth and repair of muscles. Every meal should aim to contain lean protein sources such fish, poultry, eggs, beans, lentils, and dairy products.

Carbohydrates: Carbohydrates refuel muscular glycogen stores and give exercise energy. For long-lasting energy and fiber, choose complex carbs found in whole grains, fruits, vegetables, and legumes.

Good Fats: Good fats are essential for the synthesis of hormones, the health of joints, and the absorption of nutrients. Add unsaturated fat-containing foods to your diet, such as avocados, nuts, seeds, olive oil, and fatty fish like mackerel and salmon.

When to Eat:

Pre-Workout: To give continuous energy and reduce hunger, eat a balanced breakfast with protein, carbs, and a little amount of fat 1-2 hours before working out. Steer clear of large, high-fat meals that could make working out uncomfortable.

Post-Workout: To promote muscle repair and glycogen replacement, eat a combination of carbohydrates and protein within 30 to 60 minutes of working out. Choose foods that are simple to digest, such as whole grain bread with turkey sandwiches, yogurt with fruit, or protein shakes.

Maintain Hydration:

Stay hydrated by drinking lots of water throughout the day, especially before, during, and after physical activity. Dehydration might make it harder to recover and perform poorly. Try to consume 8 to 10 glasses of water or more if you exercise vigorously or it's very hot outside.

Pre-exercise Fueling:

Before doing out, choose carbs that are easy to digest and provide you a quick energy boost, like bananas, dates, energy bars, or sports beverages. Mix a modest amount of protein with carbs to boost your muscles and provide long-lasting energy.

Nutrition for Recovery:

Prioritize eating foods high in protein and carbs after working out to aid in muscle regeneration and restore glycogen levels. To maximize recuperation, try to have a 3:1 or 4:1 ratio of carbs to protein. Add in carbs like sweet potatoes, rice, quinoa, or fruit, as well as high-quality protein sources like chicken, tofu, Greek yogurt, or protein shakes.

Keep an eye on portion sizes:

Be mindful of serving sizes to prevent overindulging or undernutrition. To determine the right serving sizes of protein, carbs, and fats, use your hand or a measuring cup. When deciding how much to eat and when to quit, pay attention to your body's signals of hunger and fullness.

Include Foods High in Nutrients:

To promote general health and fitness, choose nutrient-dense foods that are high in vitamins, minerals, and antioxidants. Your meals and snacks should include a range of vibrant fruits and vegetables, whole grains, lean meats, and healthy fats.

Arrange and Get Ready for Meals:

To make sure you always have wholesome options on hand when you need them, plan and prepare your meals in advance. Grain blends, veggies, and protein sources can be batch cooked for simple, fast meals all week long. For on-the-go fuelling, bring along portable foods like fruit, nuts, Greek yogurt, or protein bars.

Pay Attention to Your Body:

Consider the effects of various foods on your mood before, during, and after exercise. To determine what is ideal for your body and performance objectives, experiment with timing, portion amounts, and dietary selections. Adapt your nutrition plan to your unique requirements and dietary choices.

You may optimize the advantages of exercise, improve recuperation, and fuel your efforts by adjusting your nutrition to support your fitness goals. Make an effort to eat a balanced diet that will support your active lifestyle and advance general health and well-being by giving you enough energy, macronutrients, and micronutrients.

Including Days for Rest and Recovery

Your workout regimen must include recovery and rest days if you want to maximize results, avoid injuries, and advance general health and wellbeing. Here's how to successfully incorporate rest and recuperation days into your training regimen:

Recognize How Important Recovery Is:

Any fitness program must include recovery because it enables your body to rebuild and repair muscles, restore energy reserves, and adjust to the strain of exercise. You run the risk of overtraining, burnout, and an elevated chance of injury if you don't get enough rest.

Plan Dedicated Rest Days:

Include rest days in your weekly exercise routine to allow your body to recuperate. Depending on your level of fitness, the intensity of your workouts, and your unique recovery needs, try to get in at least one or two full rest days every week.

Pay Attention to Your Body:

Observe your body's sensations and modify your workout regimen accordingly. Take a day off or partake in gentle, low-impact exercises like yoga, stretching, or strolling if you're feeling exhausted, sore, or lethargic.

Differential Intensity:

Include in your regimen a combination of high-intensity training, moderate-intensity training, and active rest days. You may achieve your fitness goals and allow yourself enough recovery time by varying the volume and intensity of your workouts.

Incorporate Active Recuperation:

Active rehabilitation activities that enhance blood flow, mobility, and flexibility should be done during rest or recovery days. Mild exercises like swimming, cycling, yoga, or walking can aid with rehabilitation, lessen muscular discomfort, and improve general wellbeing.

Make sleep a priority:

Aim for 7 to 9 hours of good sleep each night to enhance recuperation and maximize efficiency. Hormone balance, muscle repair, and cognitive performance all depend on sleep. To enhance the quality of your sleep, establish a calming nighttime routine, reduce screen time before bed, and create a cozy sleeping space.

Refuel and hydrate:

To promote hydration and recuperation, stay hydrated throughout the day by consuming electrolyte-rich liquids and water. Eat a well-balanced diet that includes enough protein, carbs, and healthy fats to help repair and grow muscles while also replenishing energy stores.

Apply Active Recuperation Methods:

To relieve tension in the muscles, increase flexibility, and promote healing, incorporate active recovery techniques like foam rolling, massage, stretching, and mobility exercises. These methods can lessen aching muscles and help shield the body from harm.

Keep an eye on the recovery markers:

CHAPTER FOUR

Keep an eye out for important indicators of recovery, such as soreness in the muscles, exhaustion, appetite, and mood. Make any necessary adjustments to your training volume and intensity based on these indicators to determine whether you're ready to work out.

Individuals Recover Differently:

Recuperation requirements differ from person to person and can be affected by age, degree of fitness, volume of training, and lifestyle. To keep training and recovery in a healthy balance, pay attention to your body's needs.

You can increase long-term health and fitness, minimize the chance of injury, and maximize performance by including rest and recovery days in your exercise regimen. Make rest and recuperation a top priority as part of your overall fitness regimen, and keep in mind that progress is made both during and after workouts.

Monitoring Results and Modifying Objectives

Even in an hour, monitoring results and modifying objectives are crucial elements of any effective fitness regimen. In an hour-long workout regimen, you can efficiently monitor your development and modify your objectives by following these steps:

Clearly Define Your Objectives: To start your fitness journey, make sure your goals are SMART (specific, measurable, achievable, relevant, and time-bound). Having specific goals gives your workouts direction and motivation, regardless of whether your objective is to increase strength, endurance, flexibility, or general health.

Select Key Performance Indicators (KPIs): Choose important measurements or indicators that support your objectives and can be monitored on a regular basis to gauge your progress. Weight lifted, the quantity of repetitions or sets finished, the length of the workout, the distance traveled, body measurements, and subjective metrics like perceived exertion or energy levels are a few examples.

Use a Workout Journal or Fitness App: To track your progress and keep an eye on changes over time, record your workouts in a workout journal or use a fitness app. Note information about the type of exercise, sets, reps, weights, distances, and any feelings you had during the workout.Regularly go over your journal to spot trends, patterns, and places that might be better.

Track Your Progress: Establish recurring evaluations or benchmarks to track your advancement toward your objectives. The frequency of this could be weekly, bimonthly, or monthly, based on your preferences and the objectives you have in mind. To accurately assess your success, combine subjective input with objective data from your KPIs.

Goal Adjustment: Evaluate your progress on a frequent basis and be willing to make necessary adjustments based on your body's response, your results, and evolving situations. If you're hitting or surpassing your goals on a regular basis, think about creating new, harder objectives to keep pushing yourself. If you're having trouble moving forward or encountering obstacles, review your strategy and change your objectives to something more doable or practical.

Celebrate Your Successes: No matter how tiny, acknowledge and appreciate your victories and accomplishments along the road. To keep motivated and focused on your trip, employ positive reinforcement, reward yourself for reaching goals, and acknowledge your success.

Pay Attention to Your Body: Observe your body's reaction to your exercises, taking note of any soreness, exhaustion, or overtraining. Keep an eye out for any pain or discomfort and modify the volume or intensity of your training as necessary. Progress requires rest and recuperation, so give self-care first priority and pay attention to your body's signals.

Seek Advice and Support: To objectively evaluate your progress and offer advice on goal-setting and program modifications, think about getting advice from a certified fitness expert or coach. Embrace a network of friends, family, or fellow fitness fanatics who can provide accountability, inspiration, and support.

Remain Adaptive and Flexible: Remain adaptable and ready to modify your plans and objectives in response to unforeseen events, setbacks, or new chances. Accept the path of ongoing development and progress, and practice self-compassion while you strive toward your fitness objectives.

You may make the most of your one-hour workout schedule and eventually get significant and long-lasting effects by monitoring your progress on a regular basis, making necessary goal adjustments, and remaining adaptable and flexible. Recall that success is ultimately the result of persistent effort and dedication, even when growth isn't always linear.

CONCLUSION

In conclusion, with careful preparation, perseverance, and commitment, getting healthy in less than an hour a day is possible. You may maximize the little time you have available and efficiently increase your level of fitness by according to the suggestions provided in this plan. The main ideas are summarized as follows:

Effective Exercise Programs: Mix cardiovascular, strength, flexibility, and mobility exercises into your hour-long training sessions.

Prioritize Compound Exercises: To get the most out of your workout, concentrate on compound exercises that hit several muscle groups at once.High-Intensity Interval Training (HIIT): Include HIIT exercises into your routine to increase cardiovascular fitness and burn calories as quickly as possible.

Smart Nutrition: To boost energy levels, performance, and recovery, fuel your workouts with a balanced meal full of lean proteins, complex carbs, healthy fats, and lots of water.

Rest and Recovery: Give your body time to rebuild, heal, and adjust to the stress of exercise by scheduling rest days and active recovery activities into your schedule.

Pay Attention to Your Body: Observe your body's cues and modify your training, objectives, and tactics as necessary. Recall that long-term success requires consistency and that improvement takes time.

Your physical health, strength, endurance, and general well-being can all be significantly improved by adhering to these guidelines and prioritizing fitness in your everyday routine. Keep going, don't give up, and have fun on your path to a healthier, more fit version of yourself.

THE END